NOURISHING GOLDEN YEARS·

A Comprehensive Guide To Nutrition For Seniors

By

Jake Williams

notice asserts the author's ownership of this Book and specifies that no part of the book may be reproduced without permission from the publisher.

Contents

Introduction

As the global population continues to age, the importance of nutrition in promoting health and well-being among seniors has become increasingly apparent. Good nutrition is crucial for maintaining energy levels, cognitive function, and overall health, especially in older adults who face unique physiological changes and health challenges. This introduction aims to provide an overview of why nutrition is vital in older age and how understanding the aging body can help tailor nutritional practices to support a healthier, more active lifestyle.

Importance of Nutrition in Older Age

Nutrition plays a pivotal role in every stage of life, but its importance is magnified in older age due to several factors:

1. Maintaining Muscle Mass and Strength: As we age, we naturally lose muscle mass and strength, a condition known as sarcopenia. Adequate protein intake,

along with regular physical activity, is essential to slow down this process and maintain muscle function, which is crucial for mobility and independence.

2. Supporting Immune Function: The immune system weakens with age, making older adults more susceptible to infections, illnesses, and slower

recovery times. Nutrients such as vitamins C and E, zinc, and omega-3 fatty acids play significant roles in bolstering the immune system.

3. Preventing Chronic Diseases: Older adults are at higher risk for chronic conditions like heart disease, diabetes, osteoporosis, and

hypertension. A balanced diet rich in fruits, vegetables, whole grains, lean proteins, and healthy fats can help manage and even prevent these conditions.

4. Cognitive Health: Nutrition impacts brain health, influencing cognitive function and the risk of neurodegenerative

diseases such as Alzheimer's and dementia. Nutrients like omega-3 fatty acids, antioxidants, and vitamins B6, B12, and folate are vital for maintaining brain health.

5. Improving Quality of Life: Proper nutrition enhances overall well-being, energy levels, and mood. It enables older adults to stay active,

engage in social activities, and enjoy a higher quality of life.

Understanding the Aging Body

The aging process brings about numerous changes in the body that affect nutritional needs and eating habits. Understanding these changes is crucial for developing effective nutritional strategies for older adults.

1. Metabolic Changes: Metabolism slows down with age, resulting in lower energy requirements. However, the need for nutrients remains the same or even increases. This means older adults must

consume nutrient-dense foods to meet their nutritional needs without exceeding their caloric intake.

2. Digestive Changes: The digestive system undergoes several changes with age, including reduced secretion of digestive enzymes and stomach acid, which can affect the absorption of

nutrients like vitamin B12, calcium, and iron. Conditions such as constipation and gastrointestinal discomfort become more common, making fiber and adequate hydration important.

3. Sensory Changes: Taste and smell diminish with age, which can affect appetite and food choices.

Older adults might find certain foods less appealing or may lose interest in eating altogether. Enhancing the flavor of foods with herbs and spices can help make meals more enjoyable.

4. Dental Health: Dental issues, such as missing teeth, gum disease, and ill-fitting dentures, can make

chewing difficult and painful. This can lead to a preference for softer, less nutritious foods and avoidance of hard-to-chew items like fresh fruits and vegetables. Addressing dental health and providing appropriate food textures is vital.

5. Changes in Body Composition: Aging is often

accompanied by an increase in body fat and a decrease in lean muscle mass. This shift affects how the body uses and stores nutrients, making it important to focus on muscle-preserving diets rich in protein and regular strength-training exercises.

6. Psychosocial Factors: Social isolation, depression,

and loneliness can significantly impact eating habits and nutritional status. Older adults living alone or in care facilities may lack the motivation to prepare balanced meals or may experience emotional eating. Social support and community programs can help mitigate these effects.

Chapter One: Basic Nutritional Needs For Seniors

Macronutrients

Macronutrients, which include carbohydrates, proteins, and fats, are the cornerstone of any diet, providing the energy and essential components needed for various bodily functions. For seniors, maintaining an optimal balance of these macronutrients is crucial to support overall health, prevent chronic diseases, and promote vitality. This chapter delves into the specific roles and importance of each macronutrient in the diet of older adults.

- Carbohydrates

Carbohydrates are the body's primary source of energy. They are found in foods such as grains, fruits, vegetables, legumes, and dairy products. Carbohydrates can be classified into three main categories: simple sugars, starches, and fiber.

Simple Sugars: These are quickly absorbed and

provide immediate energy. However, excessive consumption of simple sugars, found in sweets, pastries, and sugary drinks, can lead to weight gain and increased risk of type 2 diabetes. Seniors should limit their intake of simple sugars to maintain a healthy weight and avoid spikes in blood sugar levels.

1. Starches: These are complex carbohydrates that break down more slowly than simple sugars, providing a more sustained energy release. Sources include whole grains like brown rice, oats, and whole wheat products. Including whole grains in the diet is beneficial for

maintaining steady blood sugar levels and providing essential nutrients such as B vitamins and iron.

2. Fiber: Fiber is a type of carbohydrate that the body cannot digest. It plays a critical role in digestive health, helping to prevent constipation, which is a common issue among

older adults. Fiber also aids in maintaining healthy cholesterol levels and controlling blood sugar levels. Excellent sources of fiber include fruits, vegetables, whole grains, legumes, nuts, and seeds. Seniors should aim for at least 25-30 grams of fiber per day.

- Proteins

Proteins are essential for the repair and maintenance of tissues, production of enzymes and hormones, and overall immune function. As we age, our bodies require adequate protein intake to prevent muscle loss, support immune health, and maintain overall strength.

1. Animal Proteins: These are complete proteins containing all nine essential amino acids. Sources include meat, poultry, fish, eggs, and dairy products. Lean meats and low-fat dairy options are preferable to reduce intake of saturated fats, which can

negatively impact cardiovascular health.

2. Plant Proteins: These are often incomplete proteins but can provide all essential amino acids when consumed in combination. Sources include beans, lentils, tofu, tempeh, nuts, seeds, and whole

grains. Plant proteins also offer additional benefits, such as fiber and antioxidants, which contribute to overall health.

For seniors, it is recommended to consume 1.0 to 1.2 grams of protein per kilogram of body weight per day to help preserve muscle mass and function. Including a variety of protein sources throughout the day ensures a balanced intake of essential amino acids and other nutrients.

- Fats

Fats are a vital part of the diet, providing energy, supporting cell growth, protecting organs, and aiding in nutrient absorption. However, the type of fats consumed is crucial to health outcomes, particularly in older adults.

1. Unsaturated Fats: These are considered heart-healthy fats and are primarily found in plant-based oils, nuts, seeds, avocados, and fatty-fish like salmon

and mackerel. Unsaturated fats can be further divided into monounsaturated and polyunsaturated fats. Both types have been shown to reduce bad cholesterol levels and lower the risk of heart disease. Omega-3 fatty acids, a type of polyunsaturated fat, are particularly beneficial for reducing inflammation and supporting brain health.

2. Saturated Fats: These fats are typically solid at room temperature and are found in animal products such as butter, cheese, and red meat, as well as in some tropical oils like coconut and palm oil.

High intake of saturated fats can raise LDL cholesterol levels, increasing the risk of heart disease. It is advisable for seniors to limit their intake of saturated fats to less than 10% of total daily calories.

3. Trans Fats: These are artificial fats created

by hydrogenating vegetable oils, making them more solid and shelf-stable. Trans fats are commonly found in processed foods, baked goods, and margarines. They are known to increase bad cholesterol (LDL) while decreasing good cholesterol (HDL), significantly raising the risk of heart disease.

Seniors should avoid trans fats as much as possible.

To ensure a healthy intake of fats, seniors should focus on incorporating more unsaturated fats into their diet while limiting saturated and trans fats. This can be achieved by choosing olive oil or canola oil for cooking, snacking on nuts and seeds, and eating fatty fish at least twice a week.

Micronutrients

Micronutrients, which include vitamins and minerals, are essential for numerous physiological functions and maintaining overall health. As people age, the need for certain micronutrients becomes more pronounced due to changes in the body, decreased nutrient absorption, and the prevalence of chronic conditions. This section explores the vital micronutrients for seniors and their specific roles in promoting health and well-being.

- Vitamins

Vitamins are organic compounds that are crucial for metabolic processes, immune function, and cell growth. Seniors must ensure they get adequate amounts of essential vitamins, as deficiencies can lead to various health issues.

1. Vitamin A: Important for vision, immune function, and skin health. It can be found in foods like carrots, sweet potatoes, and

spinach. Vitamin A deficiency can lead to vision problems and increased susceptibility to infections.

2. Vitamin B12: Essential for nerve function, red blood cell formation, and DNA synthesis. Older adults often have difficulty absorbing

B12 due to reduced stomach acid production. Good sources include meat, dairy products, and fortified cereals. Deficiency can cause anemia, fatigue, and neurological issues.

3. Vitamin C: Known for its antioxidant properties and role in

collagen synthesis, which is vital for skin and tissue repair. It also enhances immune function. Sources include citrus fruits, strawberries, and bell peppers. A deficiency can lead to scurvy, characterized by bleeding gums and weakened immunity.

4. Vitamin D: Crucial for calcium absorption and bone health. The body synthesizes vitamin D when exposed to sunlight, but seniors often have limited sun exposure and may require dietary sources or supplements. Foods rich in vitamin D include fatty fish, fortified milk, and eggs.

Deficiency can result in osteoporosis and increased fracture risk.

5. Vitamin E: An antioxidant that protects cells from damage and supports immune function. Sources include nuts, seeds, and green leafy vegetables. Deficiency is rare but can cause

nerve and muscle damage.

6. Vitamin K: Important for blood clotting and bone health. Found in green leafy vegetables like kale, spinach, and broccoli. A deficiency can lead to excessive bleeding and weakened bones.

- Minerals

Minerals are inorganic elements that play critical roles in structural and regulatory functions in the body. Key minerals for seniors include:

1. Calcium: Vital for maintaining strong bones and teeth, and essential for muscle

function and nerve signaling. Seniors are at higher risk for osteoporosis, making calcium intake crucial. Sources include dairy products, fortified plant milks, and leafy green vegetables. A deficiency can lead to bone loss and increased fracture risk.

2. Magnesium: Involved in over 300 enzymatic reactions, including those related to muscle and nerve function, blood glucose control, and blood pressure regulation. Sources include nuts, seeds, whole grains, and leafy green vegetables. A deficiency can cause muscle cramps, mental

disorders, and osteoporosis.

3. Iron: Necessary for the production of hemoglobin, which carries oxygen in the blood. Older adults are at risk of iron deficiency anemia, particularly women post-menopause. Sources include red

meat, poultry, fish, lentils, and fortified cereals. Symptoms of deficiency include fatigue, weakness, and shortness of breath.

4. Potassium: Helps regulate fluid balance, muscle contractions, and nerve signals. It also helps counteract the negative effects of

sodium on blood pressure. Sources include bananas, oranges, potatoes, and spinach. A deficiency can lead to hypertension and increased risk of stroke.

5. Zinc: Supports immune function, wound healing, DNA synthesis,

and protein production. Found in meat, shellfish, legumes, and seeds. Zinc deficiency can result in weakened immune response and slow wound healing.

6. Selenium: Acts as an antioxidant and is important for thyroid function. Sources

include Brazil nuts, seafood, and eggs. A deficiency can lead to immune dysfunction and cognitive decline.

Hydration

Hydration is a critical component of overall health, especially for older adults. Proper hydration helps maintain bodily functions, supports cognitive health, and can prevent various medical issues. As we age, our body's ability to conserve water decreases, and the sensation of thirst often diminishes. This chapter explores the importance of hydration for seniors, the physiological changes that affect hydration, signs of dehydration, and practical tips to maintain adequate fluid intake.

Importance of Hydration

Water is essential for numerous bodily functions, including:

1. Temperature Regulation*: Water helps regulate body temperature through sweating and

respiration. Proper hydration ensures that the body can effectively cool itself in hot conditions and maintain a stable internal temperature.

2. Joint and Muscle Health: Water lubricates joints and aids in muscle function. Staying hydrated can help prevent joint pain and muscle cramps, which

are common issues in older adults.

3. Digestive Health: Adequate fluid intake is necessary for proper digestion and nutrient absorption. Water helps dissolve minerals and nutrients, making them more accessible to the body. It also aids in preventing constipation by softening stools and promoting regular bowel movements.

4. Kidney Function: Hydration is crucial for kidney function, helping to flush out toxins and waste products from the blood through urine. Proper hydration reduces the risk of kidney stones and urinary tract infections, which are more common in older adults.

5. Cognitive Function: Dehydration can impact cognitive function, leading to confusion, fatigue, and impaired short-term memory. Staying hydrated is essential for maintaining mental clarity and cognitive health.

6. Circulatory System: Water is a major component of blood, and proper hydration ensures adequate

blood volume and circulation. This is important for delivering oxygen and nutrients to tissues and organs.

Physiological Changes Affecting Hydration in Seniors

Several physiological changes in older adults can affect hydration status:

1. Decreased Thirst Sensation: Aging can diminish the body's ability to sense thirst, leading to lower fluid intake. Seniors may not feel thirsty even when their body needs water.

2. Reduced Kidney Function: The kidneys' ability to concentrate urine decreases with age, resulting in higher water loss. This makes it necessary for older

adults to consume more fluids to compensate.

3. Medication Use: Many seniors take medications that can affect hydration, such as diuretics, which increase urine production, or laxatives, which can lead to fluid loss through the intestines.

4. Chronic Conditions: Conditions such as diabetes, heart disease, and hypertension can increase the risk of dehydration. For instance, high blood sugar levels in diabetes can lead to increased urine output.

5. Decreased Mobility: Reduced mobility or physical limitations can make it more difficult for seniors to access fluids regularly,

contributing to lower fluid intake.

Signs and Symptoms of Dehydration

Recognizing the signs and symptoms of dehydration is crucial for timely intervention. Common indicators include:

1. Dry Mouth and Lips: A lack of saliva production can cause a

dry, sticky mouth and cracked lips.

2. Dark-Colored Urine: Urine that is dark yellow or amber can indicate dehydration. Healthy urine should be light yellow to clear.

3. Fatigue and Weakness: Dehydration can lead to feelings of tiredness and weakness, as the body's cells are not functioning optimally.

4. Dizziness and Confusion: Low fluid levels can affect brain function, leading to dizziness, confusion, and impaired cognitive abilities.

5. Decreased Urine Output: Producing less urine than usual can be a sign of dehydration, especially if accompanied by other symptoms.

6. Skin Elasticity: Dehydrated skin may lack elasticity. A simple test is to gently pinch the skin on the back of the hand; if it does not return to its normal position quickly, it may indicate dehydration.

Practical Tips for Maintaining Hydration

Maintaining adequate hydration involves

incorporating regular fluid intake into daily routines. Here are practical tips for seniors to stay hydrated:

1. Set a Schedule: Establish a routine for drinking fluids throughout the day. For example, have a glass of water with each meal and snack.

2. Use Reminders: Use alarms, phone reminders, or notes to

remind oneself to drink water regularly, especially if the sensation of thirst is diminished.

3. Flavor Water: If plain water is unappealing, add natural flavors such as lemon, lime, or cucumber slices to make it more palatable.

4. Eat Hydrating Foods: Incorporate water-rich

foods into the diet, such as fruits (e.g., watermelon, oranges, strawberries) and vegetables (e.g., cucumbers, celery, lettuce).

5. Keep Water Accessible: Keep a water bottle or glass of water nearby at all times, especially in frequently used areas like the living room, bedroom, and kitchen.

6. Monitor Urine Color: Regularly check the color of urine to ensure it is light yellow to clear. Darker urine is a sign to increase fluid intake.

7. Choose Hydrating Beverages: In addition to water, consume other hydrating beverages like herbal teas, milk, and broths. Avoid excessive consumption of caffeinated or alcoholic

beverages, as they can have diuretic effects.

8. Stay Cool: In hot weather, stay in cool environments and use fans or air conditioning to reduce the risk of dehydration from sweating. Wear light, breathable clothing and take cool showers or baths if necessary.

9. Consult Healthcare Providers: Speak with

healthcare providers about hydration needs, especially if taking medications that affect fluid balance. They can provide personalized advice and may recommend appropriate electrolyte solutions.

10. Monitor for Signs of Dehydration: Regularly assess for signs of dehydration and take action

promptly if any symptoms are noticed.

Chapter Two: Common Nutritional Challenges In Old Age

Decreased Appetite

As people age, it is common to experience a decrease in appetite. This can significantly impact nutritional intake and overall health. Decreased appetite in older adults can be attributed to a variety of physiological, psychological, and social factors. Understanding these factors and implementing strategies to stimulate appetite and ensure adequate nutrient intake is crucial for maintaining health and preventing malnutrition in seniors.

Causes of Decreased Appetite

1. Physiological Changes:

- Taste and Smell: The senses of taste and smell diminish with age, making food less appealing. This can lead to a reduced interest in eating.

- Digestive System: Slower digestive processes and decreased production of digestive enzymes can cause feelings of fullness and discomfort, reducing the desire to eat.

- Hormonal Changes: Aging affects hormone levels, including those that regulate hunger and satiety, such as ghrelin and leptin.

- Medications: Many medications commonly prescribed to older adults, such as antidepressants, antihypertensives, and painkillers, can cause side effects like nausea, dry mouth, and altered taste, all of which can reduce appetite.

2. Chronic Illnesses: Conditions like diabetes, heart disease, kidney disease, and

gastrointestinal disorders can affect appetite and nutrient absorption.

- Depression and Anxiety: Mental health conditions are prevalent among seniors and can lead to a loss of interest in food and eating.

3. Dental Issues:

Problems such as missing teeth, dentures, gum disease, and oral pain can make chewing and swallowing difficult, reducing the enjoyment and frequency of eating.

4. Social and Environmental Factors:

- Loneliness and Isolation: Many older adults live alone, and the lack of social interaction during meals can diminish appetite.

- Economic Constraints: Limited income can restrict access to a variety of nutritious foods, leading to a monotonous diet that fails to stimulate appetite.

Impact of Decreased Appetite

Decreased appetite can lead to inadequate nutrient intake, resulting in several health complications:

1. Malnutrition**:
Insufficient intake of
essential nutrients can
lead to weight loss,
muscle wasting,
weakened immune
function, and increased
susceptibility to
infections.

2. Frailty and Muscle
Loss**: Poor nutrition
can accelerate
sarcopenia (loss of

muscle mass), leading to weakness, decreased mobility, and higher risk of falls and fractures.

3. Cognitive Decline**: Nutrient deficiencies, particularly of vitamins B12, D, and omega-3 fatty acids, can contribute to cognitive impairment and

increase the risk of dementia.

4. Chronic Disease Management**: Poor nutrition can exacerbate existing chronic conditions and hinder recovery from illness or surgery.

Strategies to Stimulate Appetite

To combat decreased appetite and ensure adequate nutrient intake, several strategies can be employed:

1. Enhancing the Eating Experience:

- Social Meals: Encouraging meals with family, friends, or in community settings can make eating a more enjoyable and stimulating experience.

- Pleasant Environment: Creating a pleasant dining environment with attractive table settings and minimizing distractions can enhance the appeal of meals.

2. **Improving Food Appeal:**

- Flavor Enhancement: Using herbs, spices, and seasonings can enhance the flavor of food, making it more appealing. Avoid excessive use of salt, which can contribute to hypertension.

- Variety and Color: Offering a variety of foods with different colors, textures, and flavors can stimulate interest in eating.

3. Small, Frequent Meals: Rather than three large meals, encourage the consumption of smaller, nutrient-dense meals and snacks throughout the day to ensure adequate calorie and nutrient intake without

overwhelming the digestive system.

4. Nutrient-Dense Foods:

Focus on nutrient-dense foods that provide essential vitamins, minerals, and protein. Examples include lean meats, dairy products, eggs, nuts, seeds, whole grains, fruits, and vegetables.

5. Liquid Nutrition:

For those who have difficulty eating solid foods, nutrient-rich liquids such as smoothies, milkshakes, and soups can be a good alternative to provide essential nutrients.

6. Oral Health Care:

Regular dental check-ups and addressing any oral health issues can make eating more comfortable and enjoyable.

7. Medication Management:

Review medications with a healthcare provider to identify any that may be affecting appetite. Adjustments or alternatives may be available to minimize side effects.

8. Physical Activity:

Engaging in regular physical activity can stimulate appetite and improve overall health. Even light exercises like walking or stretching can be beneficial.

Digestive Issues

Digestive issues are common among older adults and can significantly impact their nutritional status and overall health. As the body ages, changes in the digestive system, along with lifestyle and medical conditions, can lead to a range of gastrointestinal problems. Understanding these issues and their management is crucial for maintaining good health and quality of life in seniors.

Common Digestive Issues in Seniors

1. Constipation:

Prevalence:

Constipation is one of the most frequent digestive complaints in older adults. It is often characterized by infrequent, hard, and painful bowel movements.

<u>Causes</u>: Factors contributing to constipation include a low-fiber diet, inadequate fluid intake, physical inactivity, and certain medications (e.g., opioids, antacids containing calcium or aluminum, and iron supplements).

<u>Management</u>: Increasing dietary fiber intake (fruits,

vegetables, whole grains), drinking plenty of fluids, and engaging in regular physical activity can help alleviate constipation. Over-the-counter laxatives may be used occasionally, but prolonged use should be under medical supervision.

2. Gastroesophageal
   Reflux Disease (GERD):

<u>Prevalence:</u> GERD, commonly known as acid reflux, occurs when stomach acid flows back into the esophagus, causing heartburn and other symptoms.

<u>Causes:</u> Contributing factors include weakening of the lower esophageal sphincter, obesity, hiatal hernia, and certain foods (e.g., spicy foods, citrus, chocolate, caffeine).

<u>Management:</u> Lifestyle modifications, such as eating smaller, more frequent meals, avoiding trigger foods, not lying down immediately after eating, and maintaining a healthy weight, can help manage GERD. Medications like antacids, H2 blockers, and proton pump inhibitors may also be prescribed.

3. Diverticulosis and Diverticulitis:

<u>Prevalence:</u>

Diverticulosis is a condition where small pouches (diverticula) form in the colon wall. When these pouches become inflamed or infected, it is referred to as diverticulitis.

<u>Causes:</u> Low fiber intake is a significant risk

factor for developing diverticulosis.

<u>Management</u>: A high-fiber diet can help prevent diverticulosis. For diverticulitis, treatment may include antibiotics, a liquid diet during flare-ups, and in severe cases, surgery.

4. Irritable Bowel Syndrome (IBS):

<u>Prevalence</u>: IBS is a functional gastrointestinal disorder characterized by abdominal pain, bloating, and altered bowel habits (diarrhea, constipation, or both).

<u>Causes</u>: The exact cause of IBS is unknown, but it is believed to involve a combination of gut-brain interaction, gut motility issues, and hypersensitivity.

Management: Dietary changes, such as following a low-FODMAP diet, managing stress, and using medications to manage symptoms, can help control IBS.

5. Swallowing Difficulties (Dysphagia):

Prevalence: Dysphagia is common in older adults and can result from neurological conditions (e.g., stroke, Parkinson's disease), muscle disorders, or structural abnormalities in the throat.

Causes: Dysphagia can lead to choking, aspiration (food entering the airway), and malnutrition.

Management: Swallowing therapy with a speech-language pathologist, modifying food textures, and using swallowing aids can help manage dysphagia.

Impact of Digestive Issues on Nutrition

Digestive issues can have a significant impact on nutrition and overall health in seniors:

1. Nutrient Absorption: Conditions like celiac disease, Crohn's disease, and chronic pancreatitis can impair the absorption of nutrients, leading to deficiencies in vitamins, minerals, and other essential nutrients.

2. Appetite and Food Intake: Symptoms such as pain, bloating, and

nausea can reduce appetite and lead to inadequate food intake, further exacerbating nutritional deficiencies.

3. Weight Loss: Chronic digestive issues can result in unintentional weight loss and muscle wasting, contributing to frailty and

decreased physical function.

Strategies to Manage Digestive Issues

1. Dietary Modifications:

- Fiber: Increasing fiber intake can help with constipation and diverticulosis, but it should be done gradually to avoid gas and bloating. Soluble fiber (found in oats, apples, and beans) can help manage diarrhea.

- Hydration: Drinking adequate fluids is essential for preventing constipation and maintaining overall digestive health.

- Avoiding Triggers: Identifying and

avoiding foods that trigger symptoms, such as fatty foods, spicy foods, caffeine, and alcohol, can help manage conditions like GERD and IBS.

2. Medications:

Medications may be necessary to manage symptoms of digestive conditions. These should be taken as prescribed and under the guidance of a healthcare provider.

3.Regular Physical Activity:

 Exercise can help stimulate digestion and improve bowel regularity. Even light activities, such as walking, can be beneficial.

3. Professional Support:

Consulting with a healthcare provider, such as a gastroenterologist, dietitian, or speech-language pathologist, can provide tailored advice and treatment plans for managing digestive issues.

Chronic Conditions Affecting Nutrition

Chronic conditions are prevalent among older adults and can significantly impact their nutritional status and overall health. These conditions often alter dietary needs, affect nutrient absorption, and influence food choices. Understanding the relationship between chronic diseases and nutrition is crucial for developing effective dietary strategies to manage these conditions and improve the quality of life for seniors.

Common Chronic Conditions Affecting Nutrition

1. Diabetes:

<u>Prevalence</u>: Diabetes is a widespread condition among seniors, characterized by high blood glucose levels.

<u>Nutritional Impact</u>: Managing diabetes involves careful monitoring of

carbohydrate intake to maintain stable blood sugar levels. Consuming complex carbohydrates, fiber-rich foods, and balanced meals is essential. Additionally, diabetes can affect nutrient absorption and increase the risk of deficiencies in magnesium, vitamin D, and chromium.

<u>Management</u>: A diet tailored to individual needs, focusing on low-glycemic index foods, regular physical activity, and consistent monitoring of

blood glucose levels is vital for managing diabetes.

2. Heart Disease:

<u>Prevalence</u>: Heart disease remains a leading cause of death among older adults.

<u>Nutritional Impact</u>: Diet plays a significant role in managing heart disease. Saturated fats, trans fats, and high sodium intake should be limited to reduce the risk of hypertension, high cholesterol, and atherosclerosis. A diet rich

in fruits, vegetables, whole grains, lean proteins, and healthy fats (such as those found in fish, nuts, and olive oil) is recommended.

<u>Management</u>: Adopting a heart-healthy diet, engaging in regular physical activity, and maintaining a healthy weight are essential strategies for managing heart disease.

3. Chronic Kidney Disease (CKD):

<u>Prevalence</u>: CKD is common among seniors and can progress to end-stage renal disease, requiring dialysis or transplantation.

<u>Nutritional Impact</u>: CKD affects the body's ability to filter waste and balance fluids, electrolytes, and nutrients. Managing protein intake is crucial to reduce kidney strain. Sodium, potassium, and phosphorus levels must be monitored and adjusted as needed. Fluid intake may also need

to be regulated to prevent fluid overload.

<u>Management</u>: A renal diet, which is often low in sodium, potassium, and phosphorus, along with controlled protein intake, is essential for managing CKD. Regular consultation with a dietitian specializing in kidney disease is recommended.

4. Osteoporosis:

<u>Prevalence</u>: Osteoporosis is characterized by

decreased bone density and an increased risk of fractures, affecting many older adults, especially women.

<u>Nutritional Impact:</u> Adequate intake of calcium and vitamin D is critical for bone health. Protein, magnesium, and vitamin K also play roles in maintaining bone density. Seniors often need to ensure they get enough of these nutrients through diet or supplements.

Management: A diet rich in dairy products, leafy green vegetables, and fortified foods, along with appropriate supplements, regular weight-bearing exercise, and sunlight exposure for vitamin D synthesis, is important for managing osteoporosis.

5. Chronic Obstructive Pulmonary Disease (COPD):

Prevalence: COPD is a group of lung diseases, including emphysema and chronic bronchitis, that cause breathing difficulties.

- **Nutritional Impact**: Maintaining proper nutrition is crucial for managing COPD, as the condition can increase energy expenditure and lead to weight loss and muscle wasting. A balanced diet with adequate calories, protein, and nutrients is essential. Eating small, frequent meals can help prevent breathlessness while eating.

<u>Management</u>: Nutritional strategies include focusing on nutrient-dense foods, avoiding gas-producing foods, and staying hydrated. Pulmonary rehabilitation and physical activity can also improve respiratory function and overall health.

6. Dementia and Alzheimer's Disease:

<u>Prevalence</u>: Cognitive decline, including dementia and Alzheimer's disease, is

common among older adults.

<u>Nutritional Impact</u>: These conditions can affect the ability to prepare and consume food, leading to weight loss and malnutrition. Ensuring adequate intake of omega-3 fatty acids, antioxidants, and other brain-healthy nutrients is important. Dysphagia (difficulty swallowing) can also complicate nutritional intake.

<u>Management:</u>

Strategies include providing nutrient-dense foods, using adaptive utensils, offering finger foods, and ensuring a calm and supportive eating environment. Caregivers play a crucial role in monitoring and assisting with nutrition.

Strategies to Manage Nutrition in Chronic Conditions

1. Individualized Nutrition Plans: Tailoring dietary recommendations to individual needs, preferences, and medical conditions is essential. Working with a dietitian can help develop personalized nutrition plans.

2. Regular Monitoring: Regularly monitoring weight, nutrient intake, and laboratory values can help detect and

address nutritional deficiencies early.

3. Education and Support: Providing education about the importance of nutrition in managing chronic conditions and offering support through healthcare providers, community programs, and support groups can empower seniors to make healthier choices.

4. Physical Activity: Encouraging regular physical activity, tailored to the individual's abilities and health status, can help manage weight, improve cardiovascular health, and enhance overall well-being.

5. Medication Management: Reviewing medications with healthcare providers to identify

any that may affect appetite or nutrient absorption and making necessary adjustments can support better nutritional status.

Chapter 3: Designing a Balanced Diet for Seniors

Daily Caloric and Nutrient Requirements

As individuals age, their caloric and nutrient needs change due to various physiological, metabolic, and lifestyle factors. Proper nutrition is essential for maintaining health, preventing chronic diseases, and enhancing the quality of life in older adults. Understanding the daily caloric and nutrient requirements for seniors is crucial for ensuring they receive adequate nutrition.

Caloric Requirements

The caloric needs of older adults depend on several factors, including age, sex, weight, height, and activity level. Generally, as people age, their basal metabolic rate (BMR) decreases, leading to lower energy requirements. However, caloric needs can vary significantly among individuals.

1. Sedentary Lifestyle: For older adults with a sedentary lifestyle

(little to no physical activity), the average caloric requirements are approximately:

- Women: 1,600 to 2,000 calories per day

- Men: 2,000 to 2,400 calories per day

2. Moderately Active Lifestyle: For those who engage in moderate physical

activity (e.g., walking, gardening), the caloric needs increase slightly:

- Women: 1,800 to 2,200 calories per day

- Men: 2,200 to 2,800 calories per day

3. Active Lifestyle: Seniors who are physically active (regular exercise or physically demanding

tasks) require more calories:

- Women: 2,000 to 2,400 calories per day

- Men: 2,400 to 3,000 calories per day

Macronutrient Requirements

Macronutrients— carbohydrates, proteins,

and fats—are essential for energy, growth, and bodily functions. The distribution of these macronutrients in the diet is crucial for maintaining health.

1. Carbohydrates: Carbohydrates should comprise 45-65% of total daily calories. They are the primary source of energy and

are found in foods like grains, fruits, vegetables, and legumes. Emphasizing complex carbohydrates (whole grains, vegetables) over simple sugars (sweets, refined grains) is important for managing blood sugar levels and providing sustained energy.

2. Proteins: Protein needs for older adults are slightly higher than for younger adults to help maintain muscle mass and support immune function. It is recommended that 10-35% of total daily calories come from protein. This translates to approximately 1.0-1.2 grams of protein per kilogram of body

weight per day. High-quality protein sources include lean meats, poultry, fish, eggs, dairy products, beans, and legumes.

3. Fats: Fats should make up 20-35% of total daily calories. Healthy fats, such as monounsaturated and polyunsaturated fats,

are preferred over saturated and trans fats. Good sources include olive oil, avocados, nuts, seeds, and fatty fish. These fats are important for brain health, hormone production, and absorption of fat-soluble vitamins.

Micronutrient Requirements

Micronutrients, including vitamins and minerals, are crucial for various bodily functions and preventing deficiencies. Some key micronutrients that require special attention in older adults include:

1. Vitamin D: Essential for bone health and immune function, vitamin D levels often decrease with age due to reduced skin synthesis and dietary intake. The recommended daily intake is 800-1,000 IU. Sources include fortified foods, fatty fish, and sunlight exposure.

2. Calcium: Critical for bone health, older adults need adequate calcium to prevent osteoporosis. The recommended daily intake is 1,200 mg for both men and women. Good sources include dairy products, fortified plant-based milks, leafy greens,

and calcium-fortified foods.

3. Vitamin B12: Vital for nerve function and red blood cell production, vitamin B12 absorption decreases with age. The recommended daily intake is 2.4 micrograms. Sources include animal

products (meat, poultry, fish, eggs, dairy) and fortified cereals.

4. Fiber: Important for digestive health and preventing constipation, fiber needs are 21 grams per day for women and 30 grams per day for men. High-fiber

foods include whole grains, fruits, vegetables, legumes, and nuts.

5. Iron: While iron needs decrease after menopause in women, it remains important for overall health. The recommended daily intake is 8 mg for both men and women.

Sources include lean meats, beans, lentils, and fortified cereals.

6. Potassium: Essential for blood pressure regulation and heart health, the recommended daily intake is 2,600 mg for women and 3,400 mg for men. Sources include fruits

(bananas, oranges), vegetables (potatoes, spinach), beans, and dairy products.

Hydration

Adequate hydration is often overlooked but is crucial for overall health. Older adults should aim to drink at least 8 cups (64 ounces) of fluids daily, primarily from water.

Hydration helps maintain body temperature, support metabolism, and prevent constipation.

The Role of Fiber

Fiber is an essential component of a healthy diet, particularly for older adults. It plays a crucial role in maintaining digestive health, preventing chronic diseases, and promoting overall well-being. Understanding the types of fiber, their benefits, and how to incorporate them into the diet is vital for ensuring seniors receive adequate nutrition.

Types of Fiber

Fiber is classified into two main types: soluble and insoluble. Both types are important for health, but they function differently in the body.

1. Soluble Fiber:

Soluble fiber dissolves in water to form a gel-like substance. It helps slow down digestion, which can aid in blood sugar control and lower cholesterol levels.

Sources: Oats, barley, legumes, apples, citrus fruits, and carrots.

2. Insoluble Fiber:

Insoluble fiber does not dissolve in water. It adds bulk to the stool and helps food pass more quickly through the digestive tract, promoting regular bowel movements.

Sources: Whole grains, nuts, seeds, beans, and vegetables like cauliflower, green beans, and potatoes.

Benefits of Fiber

1. Digestive Health:

Fiber is crucial for maintaining a healthy digestive system. It helps prevent constipation, a common issue among older adults, by adding bulk to the stool and promoting regular bowel movements.

Fiber can also help prevent diverticulosis, a condition where small pouches form in the colon wall. By keeping the digestive system moving smoothly, fiber reduces the risk of inflammation and infection in these pouches.

2. Blood Sugar Control: Soluble fiber helps regulate blood sugar levels by slowing the absorption of sugar into the bloodstream. This is particularly

beneficial for individuals with diabetes or those at risk of developing the condition.

Consuming fiber-rich foods can prevent rapid spikes and drops in blood sugar levels, contributing to better overall glucose management.

3. Heart Health:

Soluble fiber can help lower cholesterol levels by binding to cholesterol particles in the digestive system and removing them from the body. This can reduce the risk of cardiovascular disease, which is a leading cause of morbidity and mortality in older adults.

Regular consumption of fiber-rich foods is associated with lower blood pressure and reduced inflammation, further supporting heart health.

4. Weight Management:

Fiber adds bulk to the diet, which can promote feelings of fullness and satiety. This can help prevent overeating and assist in weight management, a critical factor in preventing obesity-related conditions such as type 2 diabetes and heart disease.

High-fiber foods are often less calorie-dense, allowing individuals to consume larger portions without consuming excessive calories.

Incorporating Fiber into the Diet

To ensure adequate fiber intake, older adults should aim to consume a variety of fiber-rich foods. The recommended daily intake of fiber is 21 grams for women and 30 grams for men. Here are some tips for increasing fiber intake:

1. Choose Whole Grains: Opt for whole-grain bread, pasta, and

cereals instead of refined grains.

2. Eat Fruits and Vegetables: Incorporate a variety of fruits and vegetables into meals and snacks. Leave the skin on when possible to maximize fiber content.

3. Include   Legumes**: Add beans, lentils, and peas to soups, salads, and main dishes.

4. Snack on Nuts and Seeds: Nuts and seeds are excellent sources of fiber and can be enjoyed as snacks or added to meals.

Healthy Fats vs. Unhealthy Fats

Fats are an essential part of the diet, providing energy, supporting cell growth, and aiding in the absorption of vitamins. However, not all fats are created equal. Understanding the difference between healthy and unhealthy fats is crucial for maintaining good health, particularly for older adults who may be managing chronic health conditions.

Types of Fats

1. Healthy Fats:

- Monounsaturated Fats:

These fats are liquid at room temperature and are known to reduce bad cholesterol levels (LDL) and increase good cholesterol levels (HDL).

<u>Sources</u>: Olive oil, canola oil, peanut oil, avocados, and nuts such as almonds, hazelnuts, and pecans.

- Polyunsaturated Fats:

These fats are also liquid at room temperature and include omega-3 and omega-6 fatty acids, which are essential fats that the body cannot produce on its own.

<u>Sources</u>: Fatty fish (salmon, mackerel, sardines), flaxseeds, chia seeds, walnuts, and sunflower oil.

2. Unhealthy Fats:

- Saturated Fats:

These fats are typically solid at room temperature and can raise total cholesterol levels, increasing the risk of heart disease and stroke.

<u>Sources</u>: Red meat, butter, cheese, and other full-fat dairy products, as well as tropical oils like coconut oil and palm oil.

- Trans Fats:

These are artificial fats created through the process of hydrogenation, which makes liquid oils solid at room temperature. Trans fats significantly increase the risk of heart disease by raising LDL cholesterol and lowering HDL cholesterol.

<u>Sources</u>: Processed foods, baked goods, snack foods, margarines, and fried fast foods.

Health Benefits of Healthy Fats

1. Heart Health:

Consuming healthy fats, especially omega-3 fatty acids, helps reduce inflammation, lower blood pressure, and decrease the risk of cardiovascular disease. Omega-3s are particularly beneficial for their anti-inflammatory properties.

2. Cognitive Function:

Healthy fats are crucial for brain health. Omega-3 fatty acids, found in fatty fish and flaxseeds, have been shown to reduce the risk of cognitive decline and dementia, common concerns among older adults.

3. Nutrient Absorption: Fats help in the absorption of fat-soluble vitamins A, D,

E, and K. These vitamins play vital roles in vision, bone health, immune function, and blood clotting.

Risks of Unhealthy Fats

1. Heart Disease:

Diets high in saturated and trans fats can lead to the buildup of plaque in the arteries, increasing the risk of heart attacks and strokes.

2. Inflammation:

Unhealthy fats contribute to inflammation in the body, which is linked to various chronic diseases, including arthritis, diabetes, and some cancers.

3. Weight Gain:

Foods high in unhealthy fats are often calorie-dense

and can contribute to weight gain, obesity, and associated metabolic disorders.

Practical Tips for Reducing Unhealthy Fats and Increasing Healthy Fats

1. Choose Healthier Oils:

Use olive oil, canola oil, or sunflower oil instead of

butter, lard, or shortening for cooking and baking.

2. Incorporate Fatty Fish:

Aim to eat fatty fish like salmon, mackerel, or sardines at least twice a week to boost omega-3 intake.

3. Snack Wisely:

Replace snacks high in unhealthy fats, such as chips and cookies, with healthier options like nuts, seeds, and fresh fruits.

4. Read Food Labels:

Avoid processed foods that contain trans fats by checking for "partially hydrogenated oils" on ingredient lists.

5. Limit Red Meat:

Opt for lean cuts of meat and reduce consumption of red and processed meats. Consider plant-based protein sources such as beans, lentils, and tofu.

Chapter 4: Special Dietary Considerations

Managing Diabetes

Diabetes is a chronic condition characterized by high blood sugar levels (glucose) due to either insufficient insulin production or ineffective use of insulin by the body. For seniors, managing diabetes requires careful attention to diet, physical activity, medication adherence, and regular monitoring of blood glucose levels. Proper management is crucial to prevent complications and maintain overall health.

Understanding Diabetes

Diabetes can be categorized into different types, with

Type 2 diabetes being the most common among older adults. In Type 2 diabetes, the body either becomes resistant to insulin or doesn't produce enough insulin to maintain normal blood sugar levels. This can lead to serious health complications such as heart disease, stroke, kidney disease, nerve damage, and vision problems.

Dietary Recommendations

1. Carbohydrate Management:

Carbohydrates directly affect blood glucose levels, so managing carbohydrate intake is critical. Seniors with diabetes should focus on consuming complex carbohydrates that are high in fiber and have a lower glycemic index to help stabilize blood sugar levels.

<u>Sources</u>: Whole grains (brown rice, whole wheat bread), legumes (beans, lentils), fruits, and vegetables.

2. Protein and Fat Intake:

Including lean proteins (such as chicken, fish, tofu) and healthy fats (like olive oil, avocado, nuts) in meals can help stabilize blood sugar levels and provide sustained energy.

Portion Control: Seniors should practice portion control to manage calorie intake and prevent weight gain, which can exacerbate diabetes symptoms.

3. Fiber-Rich Foods:

Fiber helps regulate blood sugar levels by slowing

down the absorption of glucose and promoting a feeling of fullness. It also supports digestive health.

Sources: Whole grains, fruits, vegetables, nuts, and seeds.

Physical Activity

Regular physical activity is beneficial for managing diabetes by improving insulin sensitivity, lowering blood sugar levels, and promoting overall cardiovascular health. Seniors should aim for at least 150 minutes of moderate-intensity aerobic activity per week, such as brisk walking, swimming, or cycling. Strength training exercises, involving major muscle groups, should also be included at least twice a week.

Medication Adherence

Many seniors with diabetes may require medications, such as oral medications or insulin injections, to manage their blood sugar levels effectively. It's crucial to follow healthcare provider's recommendations regarding medication dosage, timing, and monitoring for any side effects or interactions with other medications.

Blood Glucose Monitoring

Regular monitoring of blood glucose levels is essential for managing diabetes. Seniors should follow their healthcare provider's instructions for testing frequency and target blood sugar ranges. Monitoring helps identify patterns and allows for adjustments in diet, medication, or physical activity to maintain stable blood sugar levels.

Lifestyle Modifications

1. Smoking Cessation: Smoking increases the

risk of complications associated with diabetes, such as heart disease and circulation problems. Quitting smoking can improve overall health and reduce these risks.

2. Stress Management: Chronic stress can affect blood sugar levels. Techniques such

as deep breathing, meditation, yoga, and engaging in hobbies or social activities can help manage stress effectively.

Regular Healthcare Visits

Seniors with diabetes should schedule regular check-ups with healthcare providers, including diabetes specialists, to monitor their condition, assess complications, and adjust treatment plans as necessary. These visits may also include screenings for other health issues related to diabetes, such as eye exams and foot checks.

Heart-Healthy Eating

Heart-healthy eating is crucial for seniors to maintain cardiovascular health, reduce the risk of heart disease, and manage existing conditions such as hypertension and high cholesterol. A balanced diet rich in nutrient-dense foods can significantly impact heart health by lowering cholesterol levels, controlling blood pressure, and supporting overall well-being.

Key Principles of Heart-Healthy Eating

1. Emphasis on Whole Foods:

Whole foods, such as fruits, vegetables, whole grains, lean proteins, and healthy fats, should form the foundation of a heart-healthy diet. These foods are rich in vitamins, minerals, fiber, and antioxidants that support heart health and overall vitality.

2. Limit Saturated and Trans Fats:

Saturated fats and trans fats increase cholesterol levels and contribute to plaque buildup in the arteries, increasing the risk of heart disease and stroke. These fats are commonly found in red meat, full-fat dairy products, processed foods, and baked goods.

<u>Healthy Alternatives:</u> Replace saturated fats with unsaturated fats, such as those found in olive oil, avocados, nuts, and fatty fish like salmon and mackerel. Avoid trans fats by checking food labels and

opting for products with zero trans fats.

3. Choose Heart-Healthy Proteins:

Opt for lean proteins that are low in saturated fat, such as skinless poultry, fish, beans, lentils, tofu, and legumes. These protein sources provide essential nutrients without contributing to elevated cholesterol levels.

4. Include Omega-3 Fatty Acids:

Omega-3 fatty acids, particularly EPA and DHA, are beneficial for heart health as they help lower triglyceride levels, reduce inflammation, and support optimal heart function. Sources include fatty fish (salmon, sardines, trout), flaxseeds, chia seeds, and walnuts.

5. Reduce Sodium Intake:

Excessive sodium intake can contribute to high blood pressure, a major risk factor for heart disease. Seniors should aim to limit sodium consumption by avoiding processed foods, canned soups, salty snacks, and restaurant meals.

Flavor Alternatives: Use herbs, spices, lemon juice, and vinegar to add flavor to meals instead of salt.

6. Monitor Portion Sizes:

Controlling portion sizes helps manage calorie intake and maintain a healthy weight, which is essential for heart health. Use smaller plates and avoid oversized servings to prevent overeating.

7. Eat Fiber-Rich Foods:

Fiber supports heart health by lowering cholesterol levels, promoting healthy digestion, and aiding in weight management. Include plenty of fruits, vegetables, whole grains, nuts, seeds, and legumes in the diet to meet daily fiber needs.

Practical Tips for Seniors

1. Meal Planning: Plan meals ahead to incorporate a variety of heart-healthy foods. Include colorful vegetables, whole grains, and lean proteins in each meal.

2. Healthy Cooking Methods: Use cooking methods such as baking, grilling, steaming, and sautéing with healthy oils instead of frying. This reduces added fats and calories.

3. Hydration: Stay hydrated by drinking

plenty of water throughout the day. Proper hydration supports cardiovascular health and helps maintain optimal blood circulation.

4. Limit Alcohol: If alcohol is consumed, do so in moderation. Excessive alcohol

intake can increase blood pressure and contribute to heart disease risk.

5. Regular Exercise: Combine a heart-healthy diet with regular physical activity to enhance cardiovascular health, maintain weight, and

improve overall well-being.

6. Consultation with Healthcare Providers: Seniors with existing heart conditions or concerns should consult healthcare providers, including registered dietitians, for personalized dietary

recommendations and ongoing support.

Bone Health: Calcium and Vitamin D

Maintaining strong and healthy bones is essential for seniors to prevent osteoporosis and fractures. Calcium and vitamin D play critical roles in bone health, supporting bone density and strength. Seniors, especially women post-menopause and individuals at higher risk of bone-related conditions, should prioritize adequate intake of these nutrients through diet and supplementation.

Importance of Calcium

Calcium is a mineral that is vital for building and maintaining strong bones and teeth. As people age, bone density naturally decreases, making bones more fragile and susceptible to fractures. Adequate calcium intake helps offset this loss and supports overall skeletal health.

1. Recommended Daily Intake:

For adults aged 51 and older, the recommended daily intake of calcium is 1,200 mg. Women over 50 and men over 70 may require slightly higher amounts due to increased bone loss risk.

2. Food Sources:

Good food sources of calcium include dairy products such as milk, yogurt, and cheese. Non-dairy sources include fortified plant-based milks (soy, almond), tofu, sardines with bones, leafy green vegetables (kale, broccoli), and almonds.

3. Supplementation:

Seniors who cannot meet their calcium needs through diet alone may consider calcium supplements. It's important to choose supplements that provide calcium citrate or carbonate, which are more easily absorbed.

4. Absorption Factors:

Vitamin D plays a crucial role in calcium absorption. Without sufficient vitamin D, the body cannot effectively absorb calcium from the digestive tract, even if dietary intake is adequate.

Role of Vitamin D

Vitamin D is a fat-soluble vitamin that supports calcium absorption, bone mineralization, and overall bone health. It is synthesized in the skin upon exposure to sunlight and can also be obtained through dietary sources and supplements.

1. Recommended Daily Intake:

For adults aged 51 to 70, the recommended daily intake of vitamin D is 600 IU (International Units). For those over 70, it increases to 800 IU.

2. Sunlight Exposure:

Sunlight is a natural source of vitamin D. Seniors should aim for moderate sun exposure (about 10-15 minutes on arms, hands, and face) a few times a week, preferably during midday when the sun's rays are strongest.

3. Dietary Sources:

Vitamin D can be found in fatty fish (salmon, tuna, mackerel), egg yolks, fortified dairy products (milk, yogurt), fortified cereals, and fortified plant-based milks (soy, almond).

4. Supplementation:
Due to limited sun exposure and dietary intake, many seniors benefit from vitamin D supplements, especially during winter months or if living in northern latitudes where sunlight exposure is reduced.

Maintaining Bone Health

1. Lifestyle Factors:

Engage in weight-bearing exercises such as walking, jogging, dancing, and resistance training to stimulate bone formation and maintain bone density.

2. Avoid Excessive Alcohol and Smoking:

Both alcohol consumption and smoking can contribute

to bone loss and weaken bones over time. Limiting alcohol intake and avoiding smoking supports overall bone health.

3. Regular Bone Density Testing:

Seniors at higher risk of osteoporosis or bone fractures should discuss bone density testing with healthcare providers to monitor bone health and assess the need for preventive measures or treatments.

Chapter 5: Meal Planning and Preparation

Creating a Weekly Meal Plan

Creating a weekly meal plan is an effective strategy for seniors to promote balanced nutrition, streamline grocery shopping, and maintain overall health and well-being. A well-thought-out meal plan can help ensure that seniors meet their dietary needs, manage chronic conditions, and enjoy a variety of nutritious foods throughout the week.

Benefits of Meal Planning

1. Nutritional Adequacy:

Meal planning allows seniors to ensure they are consuming a balanced diet that includes a variety of foods from all food groups. This helps meet essential nutrient requirements for optimal health and well-being.

2. Time and Cost Efficiency:

Planning meals in advance can save time and reduce stress associated with deciding what to eat each day. It also helps seniors avoid spontaneous and potentially costly food purchases or dining out.

3. Portion Control:

Seniors can better manage portion sizes and caloric intake by planning meals ahead. This promotes healthier eating habits and can support weight management goals.

4. Health Condition Management:

For seniors managing chronic conditions such as diabetes, heart disease, or osteoporosis, meal planning allows for careful consideration of dietary restrictions and preferences. It ensures consistency in meal choices that support health goals.

5. Variety and Enjoyment:

By planning meals, seniors can incorporate a variety of flavors and cuisines into their diet, making meals more enjoyable and reducing the likelihood of monotony in food choices.

Steps to Create a Weekly Meal Plan

1. Set Goals and Consider Preferences:

Start by setting nutritional goals based on individual health needs and preferences. Consider factors such as dietary restrictions, food allergies, cultural preferences, and personal taste preferences.

2. Plan Meals for the Week:

Designate specific days for planning breakfast, lunch, dinner, and snacks. Use a template or meal planning app to organize meals, ensuring a variety of foods and nutrients are included.

3. Include Nutrient-Dense Foods:

Incorporate a balance of fruits, vegetables, whole grains, lean proteins, and healthy fats into each meal. Aim for colorful plates that signify a diverse range of vitamins, minerals, and antioxidants.

4. Consider Convenience and Preparation Time:

Choose recipes and meals that are feasible to prepare

based on available time and energy levels. Opt for simple recipes, make-ahead meals, and leftovers that can be repurposed for future meals.

5. Utilize Seasonal and Sale Items:

Take advantage of seasonal produce and grocery sales to diversify meals and reduce costs. Fresh, in-season fruits and vegetables often provide optimal flavor and nutritional value.

6. Plan for Snacks and Beverages:

Include nutritious snacks such as fruits, yogurt, nuts, and whole-grain crackers between meals. Stay hydrated by incorporating water, herbal teas, or infused waters as beverage choices.

7. Create a Shopping List:

Based on the meal plan, compile a comprehensive shopping list of necessary ingredients and groceries. Organize the list by sections of the grocery store to streamline shopping trips.

8. Flexibility and Adaptability:

Allow flexibility in the meal plan to accommodate changes in schedule, unexpected events, or leftovers. Adapt recipes or meal components as needed to prevent food waste and ensure meals remain enjoyable.

Tips for Successful Meal Planning

1. Batch Cooking: Prepare larger portions of meals and freeze individual servings for future consumption.

2. Rotate Recipes: Introduce new recipes and rotate favorite

meals to maintain
variety and prevent
culinary boredom.

3. Seek Inspiration:
Explore cookbooks,
online recipes, and
culinary blogs for
inspiration and new
meal ideas.

Quick and Nutritious Recipes

Quick and nutritious recipes are invaluable for seniors seeking convenient meal options without sacrificing health or flavor. These recipes prioritize simplicity, require minimal preparation time, and incorporate wholesome ingredients to support optimal nutrition and well-being.

Benefits of Quick and Nutritious Recipes

1. Time Efficiency:

Quick recipes minimize time spent in the kitchen, making meal preparation easier and more manageable for seniors with busy schedules or limited energy.

2. Nutritional Value:

Nutritious recipes prioritize whole foods rich in essential nutrients, such as vitamins, minerals, fiber, and antioxidants. This promotes overall health and supports specific dietary needs.

3. Variety and Enjoyment:

Quick recipes offer a variety of flavors and cuisines, ensuring meals are both nutritious and enjoyable. They allow seniors to explore new dishes without extensive cooking efforts.

4. Cost-Effectiveness:

By using simple, readily available ingredients, quick recipes help seniors save money on groceries and minimize food waste. They often utilize pantry staples and seasonal produce.

5. Portion Control and Health Management:

These recipes facilitate portion control and promote balanced eating habits, which are crucial for managing weight, blood sugar levels, and overall health conditions.

Examples of Quick and Nutritious Recipes

1. Mediterranean Quinoa Salad

- Ingredients:

- 1 cup quinoa, rinsed

- 1 cucumber, diced

- 1 pint cherry tomatoes, halved

- 1/2 cup Kalamata olives, sliced

- 1/4 cup red onion, finely chopped

- 1/4 cup fresh parsley, chopped

- Feta cheese (optional)

- Dressing: 3 tablespoons olive oil, 2 tablespoons lemon juice, 1 garlic clove (minced), salt and pepper to taste

❖ Instructions:

1. Cook quinoa according to package instructions and let cool.

2. In a large bowl, combine quinoa, cucumber, tomatoes, olives, red onion, and parsley.

3. In a small bowl, whisk together olive oil, lemon juice, garlic, salt, and pepper.

4. Pour dressing over the salad and toss gently to combine. Add feta cheese if desired. Serve chilled.

2. Pan-Seared Salmon with Roasted Vegetables

- Ingredients:

- 4 salmon fillets

-    2   cups   mixed vegetables (bell peppers, zucchini, carrots), chopped

- Olive oil

- Salt and pepper to taste

-    Lemon   wedges   for garnish

❖ Instructions:

1. Preheat oven to 400°F (200°C). Line a baking sheet with parchment paper.

2. Toss mixed vegetables with olive oil, salt, and pepper. Spread evenly on the baking sheet.

3. Roast vegetables in the oven for 20-25 minutes or until tender and lightly browned.

4. While vegetables roast, season salmon fillets with salt and pepper.

5. Heat olive oil in a skillet over medium-high

heat. Add salmon fillets, skin side down, and cook for 4-5 minutes per side until golden and cooked through.

6. Serve salmon over roasted vegetables with a squeeze of fresh lemon juice.

3. Greek Yogurt Parfait

- Ingredients

- Greek yogurt (plain or flavored)

- Fresh berries (strawberries, blueberries, raspberries)

- Granola

- Honey (optional)

❖ Instructions:

1. In a glass or bowl, layer Greek yogurt, fresh berries, and granola.

2. Repeat layers until ingredients are used, finishing with a sprinkle of granola on top.

3. Drizzle with honey if desired. Serve immediately as a nutritious breakfast or snack.

Tips for Quick Meal Preparation

1. Prep Ahead: Wash, chop, and portion ingredients in advance to streamline cooking and assembly.

2. Use One-Pot or One-Pan Recipes: Minimize cleanup and cooking time by preparing meals that require fewer dishes.

3. Explore Instant Pot or Slow Cooker Meals: Utilize these appliances for hands-off cooking of soups, stews, and hearty meals with minimal effort.

4. Keep Pantry Staples: Stock pantry with canned beans, whole grains, canned

tomatoes, and spices for quick meal assembly.

Shopping Tips for Seniors

Navigating grocery shopping can pose challenges for seniors due to mobility issues, budget constraints, and dietary considerations.

Implementing effective shopping strategies can streamline the process, ensure nutritious choices, and enhance overall convenience and satisfaction.

Importance of Effective Shopping Strategies

1. Maintaining Independence:

Effective shopping strategies empower seniors to maintain independence by facilitating efficient and successful shopping trips without assistance.

2. Budget Management:

Implementing budget-friendly shopping tips helps seniors make economical choices, maximize savings, and minimize food waste.

3. Health and Nutrition:

By focusing on nutritious foods and ingredients, seniors can support overall health, manage chronic conditions, and maintain optimal well-being through their diet.

Practical Shopping Tips for Seniors

1. Plan Ahead:

Create a shopping list based on planned meals and household needs to stay organized and focused during shopping trips. List essential items first, followed by optional or supplementary items.

2. Shop During Off-Peak Hours:

Avoid crowds and long checkout lines by shopping

during quieter times, such as early mornings or weekdays. This reduces stress and allows for a more leisurely shopping experience.

3. Utilize Grocery Delivery or Pickup Services:

Take advantage of grocery delivery or pickup services offered by local supermarkets or online platforms. These services provide convenience and eliminate the need for physical shopping trips.

4. Explore Senior Discounts and Loyalty Programs:

Many stores offer discounts specifically for seniors or loyalty programs that provide savings on groceries and other essentials. Inquire about eligibility and benefits to maximize savings.

5. Read Labels and Compare Prices:

Take time to read food labels for nutritional information, ingredients, and allergens. Compare prices of similar products to make informed choices and find the best value for money.

6. Choose Nutrient-Dense Foods:

Prioritize fresh produce, whole grains, lean proteins, and low-sodium canned goods. These nutrient-dense foods support overall health and contribute to a balanced diet.

7. Consider Portion Sizes and Storage:

Opt for smaller portion sizes or pre-packaged items to minimize waste and ensure freshness. Choose foods that are easy to store and use within a reasonable timeframe.

8. Seek Assistance if Needed:

If physical limitations or health concerns make shopping challenging, consider asking a family member, caregiver, or volunteer for assistance. Many communities offer support services for seniors.

9. Stay Hydrated and Energized**:

- Carry a water bottle and have a light snack before shopping to stay hydrated and maintain energy levels throughout the trip.

Safety Considerations

1. Use Mobility Aids if Necessary:

Utilize shopping carts, walkers, or wheelchairs provided by stores to enhance comfort and mobility during shopping.

2. Be Cautious with Heavy Items:

Avoid lifting heavy bags or items that could strain muscles or joints. Seek assistance from store staff or fellow shoppers when needed.

3. Maintain Social Distancing and Hygiene Practices:

Follow current health guidelines regarding social distancing and hygiene to protect against illnesses, especially during crowded shopping periods.

Chapter 6: Supplements and Medications

When to Consider Supplements

Supplements can play a beneficial role in filling nutrient gaps and supporting overall health, especially for seniors who may have specific dietary needs or challenges. However, it's essential to approach supplement use with caution and under the guidance of healthcare professionals to ensure safety and effectiveness.

Factors Influencing Supplement Needs

1. Dietary Deficiencies:

Seniors may experience difficulty in obtaining adequate nutrients from diet alone due to reduced appetite, limited food variety, or digestive issues. Supplements can help bridge these nutritional gaps.

2. Health Conditions:

Certain health conditions, such as osteoporosis, diabetes, or vitamin deficiencies, may require higher intake of specific nutrients that cannot be met through diet alone. Supplements tailored to these needs can support treatment and management.

3. Medication Interactions:

Some medications can deplete essential nutrients or interfere with nutrient absorption. Supplements may be necessary to counteract these effects and maintain overall health.

4. Age-Related Changes:

Aging bodies may have decreased ability to absorb certain nutrients, such as vitamin B12 and vitamin D. Supplements can ensure adequate intake and prevent deficiencies associated with aging.

Signs to Consider Supplement Use

1. Persistent Fatigue or Weakness:

Feeling consistently tired or weak despite adequate rest and nutrition may indicate a need for supplements, such as iron or B vitamins, which support energy production and red blood cell function.

2. Poor Immune Function:

Frequent illnesses or prolonged recovery from infections may suggest a weakened immune system. Supplements like vitamin C, vitamin D, and zinc can strengthen immune function and support overall immunity.

3. Bone Health Concerns:

Osteoporosis or bone fractures may signal a need for calcium, vitamin D, magnesium, and vitamin K supplements to maintain bone density and strength.

4. Cognitive Decline:

Memory problems or cognitive decline associated with aging may benefit from supplements such as omega-3 fatty acids (DHA and EPA), vitamin E, and certain B vitamins that support brain health and function.

5. Chronic Conditions:

Managing chronic conditions like diabetes,

cardiovascular disease, or arthritis may require supplements that complement treatment plans and promote overall health.

Guidelines for Supplement Use

1. Consult Healthcare Provider:

Before starting any supplements, consult with a healthcare provider, preferably a registered dietitian or physician familiar with your medical history and current health status. They can assess your individual needs and recommend appropriate supplements.

2. Choose Quality Products:

Select supplements from reputable brands that undergo third-party testing for quality, purity, and potency. Look for products with USP (United States Pharmacopeia) or NSF (National Sanitation Foundation) certification.

3. Follow Recommended Dosages:

Adhere to recommended dosages provided by healthcare professionals or as indicated on supplement labels. Avoid exceeding recommended intake levels unless advised otherwise by a healthcare provider.

4. Monitor for Side Effects:

Pay attention to any adverse reactions or side effects from supplements. Discontinue use and consult a healthcare provider if you experience persistent symptoms or concerns.

5. Integrate with Balanced Diet:

Supplements should complement a balanced diet rather than replace nutritious foods. Focus on consuming a variety of whole foods rich in essential nutrients alongside supplement use.

6. Regular Review and Adjustments:

Periodically review supplement intake with healthcare providers to assess ongoing needs, adjust dosages as necessary, and ensure supplements remain beneficial and safe.

Interactions Between Food and Medications

Understanding the interactions between food and medications is crucial for seniors to ensure safe and effective treatment outcomes. Certain foods and beverages can interact with medications, affecting their absorption, metabolism, and effectiveness. Awareness of these interactions helps seniors make informed choices about their diet and medication management.

Types of Food and Medication Interactions

1. Altering Absorption: Some medications require specific conditions for optimal absorption. For example, taking certain antibiotics with dairy

products or calcium-fortified foods can reduce absorption rates, potentially compromising treatment efficacy.

2. Impact on Metabolism:

Foods and beverages can influence how medications are metabolized in the body. Grapefruit and grapefruit juice, for instance, can inhibit enzymes responsible for breaking down medications, leading to higher blood levels and potential toxicity.

3. Affecting Effectiveness:

Certain nutrients or compounds in foods can interfere with medication effectiveness. For example, high-fiber foods can bind to certain medications, reducing their absorption and effectiveness.

4. Interaction with Nutrients:

Medications may deplete essential nutrients or interfere with their absorption. For instance, diuretics can increase urinary excretion of potassium and magnesium, necessitating dietary adjustments to maintain nutrient balance.

Common Food and Medication Interactions

1. Dairy Products and Antibiotics:

Calcium-rich dairy products can reduce the absorption of antibiotics such as tetracyclines and fluoroquinolones. It's advisable to take these medications at least 2 hours before or after consuming dairy.

2. Grapefruit and Medications:

Grapefruit and grapefruit juice contain compounds that inhibit enzymes in the liver, affecting the metabolism of certain medications, including statins, calcium channel blockers, and some psychiatric drugs. Seniors should avoid grapefruit products or consult healthcare providers regarding safe consumption.

3. High-Fiber Foods and Medications:

Fiber-rich foods, while beneficial for digestion and

heart health, can interfere with the absorption of medications like levothyroxine (thyroid medication) and certain antidepressants. Administering medications separately from high-fiber meals helps mitigate these interactions.

4. Warfarin and Vitamin K:

Warfarin, an anticoagulant medication, interacts with vitamin K found in green leafy vegetables and other foods. Consistent intake of vitamin K-containing foods is crucial for maintaining stable blood clotting levels, requiring careful monitoring and adjustment of warfarin dosage.

Tips for Managing Food and Medication Interactions

1. Read Medication Labels and Inserts:

Review medication packaging and informational inserts for guidance on food interactions. Some medications include specific instructions regarding timing of administration relative to meals.

2. Consult Healthcare Providers:

Before starting new medications or making significant dietary changes, consult healthcare providers, including pharmacists and doctors. They can provide personalized advice based on individual health conditions and medication regimens.

3. Keep a Food and Medication Journal:

Maintain a record of medications taken, food consumed, and any observed reactions or changes in health. This helps identify potential interactions and facilitates discussions with healthcare providers.

4. Timing of Medication Administration:

Follow recommended guidelines for taking medications with or without food, as advised by healthcare providers. Some medications are best absorbed on an empty stomach, while others require food to minimize stomach upset.

Safe Supplement Practices

Supplements can be beneficial for seniors to fill nutrient gaps and support overall health, but safe practices are essential to ensure effectiveness and minimize potential risks. Seniors should approach supplement use cautiously, considering their individual health needs, existing medications, and potential interactions. Adopting safe supplement practices helps promote health, avoid adverse effects, and maximize the benefits of supplementation.

Guidelines for Safe Supplement Use

1. Consult Healthcare Providers:

Before starting any new supplements, seniors should consult healthcare providers, including doctors or registered dietitians. They can assess individual health needs, recommend appropriate supplements, and discuss potential interactions with medications or existing health conditions.

2. Choose Reputable Brands:

Select supplements from reputable manufacturers that adhere to quality standards and undergo third-party testing. Look for products with certifications such as USP (United States Pharmacopeia) or NSF (National Sanitation Foundation) to ensure purity, potency, and safety.

3. Follow Recommended Dosages:

Adhere to recommended dosages as indicated on supplement labels or prescribed by healthcare providers. Avoid exceeding recommended intake levels unless advised otherwise, as excessive intake can lead to adverse effects or toxicity.

4. Read Labels and Ingredients:

Carefully read supplement labels to understand ingredients, dosage instructions, and potential allergens. Avoid supplements with unnecessary additives or fillers that may not align with personal dietary preferences or health goals.

5. Monitor for Side Effects:

Be vigilant for any adverse reactions or side effects while taking supplements. Common side effects may include digestive upset, allergic reactions, or interactions with medications. Discontinue use and consult healthcare providers if symptoms persist or worsen.

6. Integrate with Balanced Diet:

Supplements should complement a balanced diet rich in whole foods. Focus on consuming nutrient-dense foods such as fruits, vegetables, lean proteins, and whole grains to provide essential nutrients alongside supplements.

7. Consider Individual Needs:

Tailor supplement choices to individual health needs and dietary habits. Seniors with specific conditions like osteoporosis may benefit from calcium and vitamin D supplements, while those with low B12 levels may require vitamin B12 supplementation.

Commonly Recommended Supplements for Seniors

1. Calcium and Vitamin D: Essential for bone health and preventing osteoporosis. Seniors often require supplementation to meet daily intake

recommendations, especially if dietary sources are inadequate.

2. Vitamin B12:

Supports nerve function, red blood cell production, and cognitive health. Seniors at risk of deficiency due to age-related factors or dietary restrictions may benefit from supplementation.

3. Omega-3 Fatty Acids:

Promote heart health, cognitive function, and joint health. Omega-3 supplements derived from fish oil or algae can provide essential fatty acids not always obtained through diet alone.

4. Multivitamins:

Provide a convenient way to supplement multiple vitamins and minerals in one formulation. Choose multivitamins specifically formulated for seniors to address age-related nutrient needs.

Tips for Safe Storage and Usage

1. Store Supplements Properly:

Keep supplements in their original containers, stored in a cool, dry place away from direct sunlight and humidity. Follow storage instructions provided on supplement labels to maintain potency and freshness.

2. Discard Expired Supplements:

Check expiration dates regularly and discard expired supplements. Expired products may lose effectiveness or pose health risks if consumed beyond their shelf life.

3. Keep Records and Track Usage:

Maintain a record of supplements taken, dosages, and any observed effects. Tracking usage helps monitor adherence to recommended intake levels and facilitates discussions with healthcare providers.

Chapter 7: Overcoming Barriers to Healthy Eating

Financial Constraints

Seniors often face unique financial challenges due to retirement, fixed incomes, healthcare costs, and potentially limited access to additional sources of income. These constraints can significantly impact their ability to meet essential needs and maintain a comfortable lifestyle.

Healthcare Costs

1. Medication Expenses: Prescription medications are often a significant financial burden for seniors, especially those managing chronic conditions. High medication costs may lead to

medication non-adherence or choosing between essential medications and other necessities.

2. Medical Services and Insurance:

Medicare coverage typically assists with healthcare costs for seniors, but out-of-pocket expenses, including copayments, deductibles, and services not covered by insurance, can accumulate quickly. This can strain limited budgets and affect access to necessary medical care.

Daily Living Expenses

1. Housing and Utilities:

Housing costs, including rent, mortgage payments, property taxes, and utilities, can consume a large portion of a senior's income. Rising utility costs and maintenance expenses may necessitate budget adjustments.

2. Food and Nutrition:

Seniors may face challenges affording nutritious food due to fixed incomes and rising food prices. Food insecurity can impact health outcomes and exacerbate existing health conditions.

3. Transportation:

Costs associated with transportation, including fuel, vehicle maintenance, or public transportation fees, can strain budgets. Limited mobility options may restrict access to essential services and social activities.

Quality of Life Considerations

1. Social and Recreational Activities:

Engaging in social activities and recreational pursuits may become financially challenging for seniors. Costs associated with memberships, outings, or cultural events may be prohibitive, limiting opportunities for social interaction and mental stimulation.

2. Home Modifications and Assistive Devices:

Aging in place often requires home modifications and assistive devices to enhance safety and accessibility. However, these modifications can be costly, posing financial barriers for seniors wishing to remain independent at home.

Coping Strategies and Support Resources

1. Budgeting and Financial Planning:

Seniors can benefit from budgeting tools and financial planning services to manage expenses effectively. Seeking assistance from financial advisors or senior services agencies can provide guidance on budget allocation and resource management.

2. Utilizing Community Resources**:

Local community centers, senior centers, and

nonprofit organizations often offer support programs, including food assistance, transportation services, and financial counseling. These resources help seniors navigate financial challenges and access essential services.

3. Prescription Assistance Programs:

Pharmaceutical companies, government agencies, and nonprofit organizations administer prescription assistance programs that provide discounts or free medications to eligible seniors. Researching available programs and eligibility criteria can help reduce medication costs.

4. Advocating for Policy Changes:

- Seniors and advocacy groups can advocate for policy changes aimed at improving financial assistance programs, expanding healthcare coverage, and reducing prescription drug costs. Active involvement in community initiatives and legislative advocacy can

drive systemic changes
benefiting seniors.

Limited Mobility and Access to Food

Seniors experiencing limited mobility encounter various obstacles that affect their ability to obtain nutritious food, leading to potential health risks and diminished quality of life.

Transportation Barriers

1. Difficulty in Grocery Shopping:

Seniors with limited mobility may find it challenging to physically navigate grocery stores, push shopping carts, or carry heavy bags. Lack of accessible transportation options further restricts their ability to visit supermarkets regularly.

2. Dependence on Others

Reliance on family members, caregivers, or community services for transportation to grocery stores can be inconsistent or unavailable, leaving seniors dependent on others for food access.

Access to Nutritious Food

1. Limited Availability of Healthy Options:

Seniors residing in areas with limited access to grocery stores or markets offering fresh produce and nutritious foods may rely on convenience stores or fast food establishments, which often lack healthy options.

2. Financial Constraints:

Fixed incomes and healthcare expenses may restrict seniors' purchasing power, affecting their ability to afford nutritious foods. This can lead to compromised dietary quality and nutrient intake.

Physical Limitations

1. Difficulty in Meal Preparation:

Seniors with mobility issues may struggle with meal preparation tasks such as chopping vegetables, standing for extended periods, or using kitchen appliances safely. This can discourage cooking at home and lead to reliance on pre-packaged or convenience foods that are often less nutritious.

2. Risk of Malnutrition:

Inadequate access to nutritious food increases the risk of malnutrition among seniors with limited mobility. Malnutrition can exacerbate existing health conditions, weaken immune function, and impair overall well-being.

Strategies to Improve Access to Food for Seniors with Limited Mobility

1. Home Delivery Services:

Utilizing grocery delivery services offered by supermarkets, local markets, or online platforms allows seniors to shop for groceries from home. Delivery options ensure access to a variety of fresh produce, pantry staples, and specialty items without leaving the house.

2. Meal Delivery Programs:

Meal delivery services and programs cater specifically to seniors, providing ready-to-eat meals or meal kits that require minimal preparation. These services offer nutritious meal options tailored to dietary preferences and health needs.

3. Community Support and Resources:

Engaging with community organizations, senior centers, or religious groups can connect seniors with volunteer programs offering grocery shopping assistance, meal delivery, or transportation services.

4. Accessible Transportation Options:

Advocating for and utilizing accessible transportation services, such as senior shuttle programs, paratransit services, or rideshare options equipped with wheelchair accessibility, enhances mobility and facilitates grocery shopping trips.

5. Nutrition Education and Support:

Providing nutrition education workshops and resources for seniors with limited mobility empowers them to make informed dietary choices. Guidance on meal planning, budgeting for nutritious foods, and adapting recipes to physical capabilities promotes healthier eating habits.

6. Home Modifications:

Adapting home environments with assistive devices, ergonomic kitchen tools, and safety modifications improves independence in meal preparation and enhances access to nutritious food.

Psychological Factors: Loneliness and Depression

To discuss "Psychological Factors: Loneliness and Depression" in Chapter 7, it's essential to explore how these issues impact seniors and strategies to address them within the context of aging and health.

Impact of Loneliness and Depression on Seniors

Loneliness and depression are prevalent psychological factors among seniors that can significantly affect their mental health, quality of life, and overall well-being.

Loneliness

1. Social Isolation:

Seniors may experience social isolation due to factors such as retirement, loss of loved ones, physical health limitations, or geographic distance from family and friends. This isolation contributes to feelings of loneliness and emotional distress.

2. Health Consequences:

Prolonged loneliness is associated with adverse health outcomes, including increased risk of cardiovascular disease, cognitive decline, weakened immune function, and accelerated aging. It also correlates with higher mortality rates among older adults.

Depression

1.   Symptoms and Impact:

Depression in seniors may present differently from younger adults, with symptoms such as persistent sadness, loss of interest in activities, sleep disturbances, changes in appetite, fatigue, and feelings of worthlessness. Untreated depression can impair daily functioning and exacerbate physical health conditions.

2.   Risk Factors:

Risk factors for depression in seniors include chronic health conditions, chronic pain, medication side effects, bereavement, social isolation, financial stress, and cognitive decline. These factors contribute to the vulnerability of older adults to developing depressive symptoms.

Strategies to Address Loneliness and Depression in Seniors

1. Social Engagement Programs: Community-based programs, senior centers, and

recreational activities provide opportunities for social interaction, peer support, and engagement in meaningful activities. These programs combat loneliness by fostering connections and reducing social isolation.

2. Technology and Virtual Connectivity:

Seniors can benefit from technology platforms, social media, video calls, and online communities to stay connected with family, friends, and support networks. Virtual interactions offer a convenient way to maintain relationships and combat feelings of loneliness.

3. Counseling and Therapy: Psychotherapy, cognitive behavioral therapy (CBT), or counseling sessions tailored for seniors address underlying emotional issues, provide coping strategies, and promote emotional resilience. Therapists

help seniors explore feelings of loneliness, manage depression symptoms, and improve overall mental well-being.

4. Support Groups and Peer Counseling:

Participation in support groups for seniors experiencing similar life transitions, health challenges, or loss provides a sense of belonging, validation, and emotional support. Peer counseling allows seniors to share experiences, receive guidance, and build supportive relationships.

5. Physical Activity and Wellness Programs:

Regular exercise, yoga, tai chi, or mindfulness

practices promote mental and physical well-being. These activities reduce stress, improve mood, enhance cognitive function, and increase social interaction within structured group settings.

6. Medical Evaluation and Treatment:

Consulting healthcare providers for

comprehensive assessments and management of physical health conditions, medication reviews, and treatment adjustments help mitigate factors contributing to depression. Pharmacological interventions and psychiatric consultations may be considered for severe depressive symptoms.

Chapter 8: Practical Tips for Caregivers

Encouraging Healthy Eating Habits

Encouraging healthy eating habits among seniors is crucial for promoting overall well-being, managing chronic conditions, and maintaining quality of life. Adopting nutritious dietary practices supports physical health, enhances energy levels, and contributes to cognitive function. Here's a comprehensive approach to promoting healthy eating habits for seniors:

Importance of Healthy Eating for Seniors

1. Nutritional Needs:

Seniors have unique nutritional requirements

influenced by age-related changes, health conditions, and medication use. A balanced diet rich in essential nutrients supports immune function, bone health, and cardiovascular health.

2. Disease Prevention and Management:

Healthy eating habits reduce the risk of chronic

diseases such as diabetes, hypertension, and heart disease. Nutrient-dense foods support disease management and improve overall health outcomes.

3. Energy and Vitality:

Proper nutrition enhances energy levels, supports muscle strength, and promotes independence in daily activities. Seniors who prioritize healthy eating often experience improved mobility and overall vitality.

Strategies to Encourage Healthy Eating Habits

1.   Education and Awareness:

Provide nutrition education workshops, seminars, or one-on-one consultations for seniors. Focus on understanding dietary guidelines, portion control, reading food labels, and making informed food choices.

2.   Promote Nutrient-Dense Foods:

Emphasize the importance of consuming a variety of fruits, vegetables, whole grains, lean proteins, and low-fat dairy products. Encourage seniors to incorporate colorful produce and fiber-rich foods into their meals.

3.   Meal Planning and Preparation:

Offer resources and guidance on meal planning, grocery shopping, and simple meal preparation techniques. Encourage seniors to plan balanced meals that include protein, carbohydrates, healthy fats, and vitamins.

4. Adapt Recipes and Preferences:

Respect individual dietary preferences, cultural traditions, and health needs when recommending recipes or meal ideas. Provide alternatives and adaptations to accommodate dietary restrictions or preferences.

5. Social Dining Opportunities:

Organize communal dining events, potluck gatherings, or cooking clubs where seniors can share meals and socialize. Social dining fosters a sense of community, enjoyment of food, and peer support for healthy eating.

6.   Incorporate Physical Activity:

Promote regular physical activity alongside healthy eating habits. Encourage seniors to engage in gentle exercises such as walking, yoga, or chair exercises to support metabolism, digestion, and overall well-being.

Practical Tips for Seniors

1. Hydration:

Emphasize the importance of staying hydrated by drinking water throughout the day. Limit sugary beverages and caffeinated drinks that may contribute to dehydration.

2. Mindful Eating:

Encourage seniors to practice mindful eating by paying attention to hunger cues, chewing food slowly, and savoring flavors. Mindfulness promotes enjoyment of meals and prevents overeating.

3. Healthy Snacking:

Recommend nutritious snack options such as fresh fruits, yogurt, nuts, or whole-grain crackers. Encourage seniors to choose snacks that provide sustained energy and support nutritional goals.

4. Family and Caregiver Involvement:

Engage family members, caregivers, and support

networks in promoting healthy eating habits for seniors. Collaborate on meal planning, grocery shopping, and creating a supportive eating environment.

Adapting Meals for Different Health Conditions

As individuals age, they often encounter various health conditions that necessitate tailored dietary adjustments. Proper meal adaptation can help manage symptoms, improve health outcomes, and enhance quality of life for seniors with specific health needs. Here are strategies for adapting meals to address common health conditions among seniors:

❖ Diabetes

1. Carbohydrate Management:

Monitoring carbohydrate intake is crucial for managing blood glucose levels. Encourage the consumption of complex carbohydrates such as whole grains, vegetables, and legumes, which provide steady energy release.

2. Glycemic Index Awareness:

Teach seniors to choose foods with a low glycemic index (GI) to prevent spikes in blood sugar. Examples include whole grains, nonstarchy vegetables, and most fruits.

3. Balanced Meals:

Emphasize balanced meals that include lean protein, healthy fats, and fiber. Proteins and fats help slow down the absorption of carbohydrates, stabilizing blood sugar levels.

1. Low-Sodium Diet:

Reducing sodium intake helps manage blood pressure. Encourage the use of herbs and spices instead of salt for flavoring, and avoid processed foods high in sodium.

2. Healthy Fats:

Incorporate sources of healthy fats such as avocados, nuts, seeds, and fatty fish like salmon. These fats can help reduce inflammation and support cardiovascular health.

3. Fiber-Rich Foods:

Promote the intake of soluble fiber from foods like oats, beans, and fruits, which can help lower cholesterol levels and improve heart health.

❖ Hypertension

1. DASH Diet:

The Dietary Approaches to Stop Hypertension (DASH) diet is beneficial for managing high blood pressure. It emphasizes fruits, vegetables, whole grains, lean proteins, and low-fat dairy products.

2. Potassium-Rich Foods:

Foods high in potassium, such as bananas, sweet potatoes, and spinach, help counteract the effects of sodium and lower blood pressure.

3. Limit Caffeine and Alcohol:

Reducing the intake of caffeine and alcohol can help maintain stable blood pressure levels.

❖ Osteoporosis

1. Calcium and Vitamin
   D:

Ensure adequate intake of calcium and vitamin D to support bone health. Include dairy products, leafy greens, fortified foods, and fatty fish in the diet.

2. Protein Intake:

Adequate protein is essential for bone repair and maintenance. Encourage lean protein sources such as poultry, fish, beans, and tofu.

3. Avoid Excessive Salt and Caffeine:

High salt and caffeine intake can lead to calcium loss. Encourage moderation in the consumption of salty foods and caffeinated beverages.

❖ Kidney Disease

1. Low-Protein Diet:

For those with advanced kidney disease, a low-protein diet may be recommended to reduce the workload on the kidneys. However, adequate protein is still necessary to prevent muscle loss.

2. Phosphorus and Potassium Management:

Limit foods high in phosphorus (such as dairy products and nuts) and potassium (such as bananas and potatoes) if necessary, based on individual health needs.

3. Fluid Intake:

Monitor and adjust fluid intake according to medical advice to prevent fluid overload.

Digestive Disorders

1. High-Fiber Diet:

For constipation or diverticulosis, a high-fiber diet including whole grains, fruits, and vegetables can promote regular bowel movements.

2. Low-FODMAP Diet:

For those with irritable bowel syndrome (IBS), a low-FODMAP diet can reduce symptoms. This involves limiting foods high in fermentable oligosaccharides, disaccharides, monosaccharides, and polyols.

3. Probiotics and Prebiotics:

Incorporating probiotic-rich foods like yogurt and prebiotic fibers like chicory root can support gut health and improve digestion.

Ensuring Safety in Food Preparation

Ensuring food safety is crucial, especially for seniors who may be more vulnerable to foodborne illnesses due to weakened immune systems and underlying health conditions. Safe food preparation practices can prevent contamination and promote health and well-being. Here are essential guidelines and practices for ensuring safety in food preparation:

Personal Hygiene

1. Hand Washing:

Wash hands thoroughly with soap and water for at least 20 seconds before and after handling food, after using the restroom, and after touching pets or garbage. Hand hygiene is critical in preventing the spread of pathogens.

2. Proper Attire:

Wear clean clothing and, if necessary, use disposable gloves when preparing food. Avoid wearing jewelry that can harbor bacteria and keep hair tied back to prevent contamination.

Kitchen Cleanliness

1. Sanitize Surface:

Regularly clean and sanitize kitchen surfaces, including countertops, cutting boards, and utensils, before and after food preparation. Use a solution of one tablespoon of bleach per gallon of water to disinfect surfaces.

2. Separate Cutting Boards:

Use separate cutting boards for raw meats, fruits, and vegetables to prevent cross-contamination. Color-coded boards can help distinguish between different types of food.

Safe Food Handling

1. Temperature Control:

Keep perishable foods refrigerated at or below 40°F (4°C) and frozen foods at or below 0°F (-18°C). Use a food thermometer to ensure cooked foods reach safe internal temperatures: 165°F (74°C) for poultry, 160°F (71°C) for ground meats, and 145°F (63°C) for whole meats and fish.

2. Thawing Foods:

Thaw frozen foods in the refrigerator, under cold running water, or in the microwave. Avoid thawing at room temperature to prevent bacterial growth.

3. Avoid Cross-Contamination:

Store raw meat, poultry, and seafood separately from other foods in the refrigerator. Use sealed containers or plastic bags to prevent juices from contaminating other items.

Proper Cooking Practices

1. Cook Thoroughly:

Ensure all foods, especially meats, are cooked thoroughly to kill harmful bacteria. Use a food thermometer to verify that foods reach their safe internal temperatures.

2. Reheat Safely:

When reheating leftovers, ensure they reach an internal temperature of 165°F (74°C) to eliminate potential bacteria. Stir foods during reheating to ensure even heating.

Storing Leftovers

1. Timely Refrigeration:

Refrigerate leftovers within two hours of cooking. Divide large portions into smaller containers for quicker cooling. Leftovers should be consumed within three to four days.

2. Labeling and Dating:

Label and date all stored foods to keep track of their freshness. Discard any food that shows signs of spoilage, such as unusual odors, colors, or textures.

Special Considerations for Seniors

1. Avoid High-Risk Foods:

Seniors should avoid high-risk foods such as raw or undercooked eggs, meats, and seafood, unpasteurized dairy products, and deli meats unless heated to steaming hot. These foods are more likely to contain harmful bacteria.

2.   Hydration and Nutrition:

Ensure that seniors stay hydrated and consume a balanced diet. Nutritional needs may vary, so it's important to tailor diets to individual health conditions and dietary restrictions.

Educating Caregivers and Seniors

1. Training and Resources:

Provide training and resources on food safety practices to caregivers and seniors. Use visual aids, checklists, and easy-tounderstand guides to reinforce key concepts.

2. Regular Monitoring:

Encourage regular monitoring of food safety practices in the kitchen. Periodic reviews and updates of safety protocols ensure continued adherence to best practices.

Chapter 9: Real-Life Stories and Testimonials

Success Stories from Seniors

Success stories from seniors who have embraced healthy eating and lifestyle changes offer valuable insights and inspiration for others facing similar challenges. These stories demonstrate the positive impact of nutrition and wellness interventions on overall health and quality of life. Here are a few examples of seniors who have successfully improved their well-being through dietary and lifestyle changes:

Martha's Journey to Managing Diabetes

Martha, a 68-year-old retiree, was diagnosed with type 2 diabetes five years ago. Initially overwhelmed by the diagnosis, she struggled with managing her blood sugar levels. With the support of her healthcare team, Martha embarked on a journey to transform her eating habits and incorporate regular physical activity into her daily routine.

1. Dietary Changes:

Martha adopted a balanced diet rich in whole grains, lean proteins, and plenty of vegetables. She learned to count carbohydrates and choose foods with a low glycemic index to keep her blood sugar stable.

2. Physical Activity:

She started walking for 30 minutes each day, gradually increasing her pace and distance. Walking became a routine part of her day, contributing to better glucose control and overall fitness.

3. Support System:

Martha joined a local diabetes support group

where she shared experiences and learned from others facing similar challenges. The camaraderie and shared knowledge were instrumental in her success.

Today, Martha's blood sugar levels are well-controlled, and she feels more energetic and confident in managing her diabetes. Her story highlights the importance of dietary modifications, physical activity, and community support in managing chronic conditions.

Robert's Heart Health Transformation

Robert, a 72-year-old widower, was diagnosed with hypertension and high cholesterol. His doctor advised him to adopt a heart-healthy diet to reduce his risk of cardiovascular disease. Initially resistant to change, Robert gradually embraced new eating habits and lifestyle adjustments.

1. Dietary Adjustments:

Robert incorporated more fruits, vegetables, whole grains, and lean proteins into his meals. He reduced his intake of red meat, processed foods, and high-sodium snacks.

2. Mindful Eating:

He started practicing mindful eating, paying

attention to portion sizes and savoring each bite. This helped him avoid overeating and make healthier food choices.

3. Physical Activity:

Robert joined a local senior exercise class that included activities like tai chi and low-impact aerobics. Regular exercise helped him lower his blood pressure and improve his cardiovascular health.

After a year of these changes, Robert's blood pressure and cholesterol levels significantly improved, and he felt more active and engaged in life. His success story underscores the impact of a heart-healthy diet and regular exercise on managing cardiovascular health.

Linda's Osteoporosis Management

Linda, a 70-year-old grandmother, was diagnosed with osteoporosis after suffering a minor fracture. Concerned about her bone health, she sought guidance on how to strengthen her bones and prevent future fractures.

1. Calcium and Vitamin D:

Linda increased her intake of calcium and vitamin D through diet and supplements, incorporating foods like dairy products, leafy greens, and fortified cereals.

2. Strength Training:

She began a strength training program designed for seniors, focusing on weight-bearing exercises to improve bone density and muscle strength.

3. Fall Prevention:

Linda made her home safer by removing tripping hazards and installing grab bars in the bathroom. She also practiced balance exercises to reduce her risk of falls.

Linda's proactive approach resulted in improved bone density and reduced her risk of fractures. Her story highlights the importance of targeted nutrition, exercise, and environmental modifications in managing osteoporosis.

THE END